JASMINE J. WILLIS

Rosacea Relief

Discover the Power of Natural Treatments and Little-Known Remedies for Stunning Results! An In-Depth Guide to Understanding Rosacea Signs, Symptoms, and Gentle Therapies That Work Wonders

Contents

Preface

In this comprehensive guide, "Rosacea Relief: Discover the Power of Natural Treatments and Little-Known Remedies for Stunning Results," delve into the world of rosacea—a chronic skin condition that manifests in the central parts of the face and often misunderstood by many. My journey began from a personal struggle and evolved into a deep academic exploration, driven by a desire to uncover the true dynamics of rosacea, from its subtle early symptoms to its more pronounced stages.

This book is born out of countless interactions with dermatologists, hours of reviewing scientific studies, and my firsthand experiences with the condition. Here, I aim to demystify rosacea by providing a clear overview of its signs, symptoms, and the myriad treatment options available—from conventional medical approaches to transformative natural remedies that have proven efficacy but remain underutilized.

Throughout the chapters, you will find practical advice tailored to managing and treating rosacea effectively, fostering a better quality of life. This guide also includes a discussion on the emotional and psychological impacts of living with rosacea, which many sufferers report as being equally challenging.

My hope is that by sharing both my professional insights and personal experiences, this book will serve as a beacon of understanding and ope for those affected by rosacea. Whether you are newly diagnosed, a long-time sufferer, or a caregiver, "Rosacea Relief" is designed to equip you with the knowledge to take control of your skin health and regain your confidence.

I

Part One

All You Need to Know About Rosacea from signs, symptoms, treatment, type, causes and medical treatment

Chapter 1

Rosacea: Signs, Symptoms and Treatment

Rosacea (pronounced "roh-ZAY-sha") is a persistent but curable skin condition that mostly affects the central face and is marked by flare-ups and remissions. Although rosacea may develop in a variety of ways and at any age, patient surveys indicate that it often appears after the age of 30 as periodic flushing or redness on the cheeks, nose, chin, or forehead. According to studies, the redness gradually becomes ruddier and more persistent, and visible blood vessels may develop. Left untreated, inflammatory bumps and pimples often appear, and in extreme instances — especially in males — the nose may become bloated and bumpy due to excess tissue. Up to half of all patients' eyes get inflamed, becoming watery or bloodshot.

Although rosacea affects all demographics and skin types, people with fair complexion who flush or blush easily are thought to be the most vulnerable. Women are more likely to be diagnosed with the disease, and males take it more seriously. There is also evidence that rosacea runs in families and may be more common in people of northern or eastern European heritage.

According to studies conducted by the National Rosacea Society

(NRS), more than 90% of rosacea patients said that their condition ha
harmed their self-confidence and self-esteem, with 41% avoiding publi
involvement or canceling social gatherings. Almost 88% of people wit
severe rosacea said that the condition had harmed their profession:
connections, and almost 51% stated they had missed work as a result c
their sickness. The good news is that more than 70% of respondents sai
that medical therapy enhanced their emotional and social well-being

While the etiology of rosacea is unclear and there is no cure, under
standing of the signs and symptoms has grown to the point that medica
treatment and lifestyle modifications may be used to treat it successfull
Individuals who feel they have rosacea should see a dermatologist o
another expert physician to get a diagnosis and suitable treatment befor
the illness progresses and interferes with everyday activities.

What Should I Look for?

Rosacea varies greatly from person to person, and in most situations
just a few of the potential signs and symptoms manifest. A consensu
committee and review panel of 28 medical professionals from across
the globe determined that at least one diagnostic symptom or two
main indicators of rosacea are required for a diagnosis.1 A variety
of secondary signs and symptoms may arise, although they are not
diagnostic.

Diagnostic Signs of Rosacea

Rosacea is diagnosed when any of the following symptoms arise.

Persistent Redness

The most frequent symptom of rosacea is persistent face redness,
which might mimic a lingering flush or sunburn.

Skin Thickening

Excess tissue on the nose may cause the skin to thicken and expand, condition known as rhinophyma. Although less prevalent, this ondition may cause facial abnormalities and decreased nasal airflow if evere.

Rosacea's most common symptoms.

Rosacea is diagnosed when two or more of the following symptoms ppear.

lushing

Many individuals with rosacea experience frequent blushing or ushing. This face redness, which might be accompanied by a feeling f heat, warmth, or burning, happens on a regular basis and is often an arly symptom of the condition.

Bumps and pimples.

Small red solid lumps or pus-filled pimples are often seen. While they esemble acne, they do not contain blackheads and may cause burning r stinging.

Visible Blood Vessels

Many rosacea patients develop large, visible tiny blood vessels called elangiectasia (pronounced "tell-ANN-jeck-TAY-zha") on their cheeks, nasal bridge, and other key face regions.

Eye discomfort.

Many rosacea sufferers have itchy, watery, or bloodshot eyes, which s known as ocular rosacea. Eyelids may become red and puffy, and styes are prevalent. Crusts and scales may form around the eyelids or lashes, and patients may see visible blood vessels along the lid margins. Severe instances may result in corneal injury and loss of visual acuity if no medical attention is offered.

Secondary signs and symptoms.

These may present as one or more of the diagnostic or main symptoms.

Burns or stings.

Burning or stinging feelings may often occur on the face. Itching or sense of tightness may also occur.

Swelling

Facial swelling, also known as edema, may occur with other rosace symptoms or on its own. Plaques, or raised red spots, may form withou affecting the surrounding skin.

Dryness

Despite worries about oily skin, the central face skin may be rough and scaly.

Rosacea symptoms may occasionally appear on the neck, chest, scalp or ears.

The signs of Rosacea are:

Facial redness and flushing. Rosacea may make your face blush more quickly. Over time, you may find that your face remains red. Depending on the skin tone, redness might be faint or seem more pink or purple.

Visible veins. Small blood vessels in the nose and cheeks burst and expand. These are also known as spider veins. They might be faint and difficult to notice depending on skin tone.

Swollen bumps. Many individuals with rosacea develop pimples on their faces that resemble acne. These pimples might include pus. They may also occur on the back and chest.

Burning feeling. The skin in the afflicted region may be heated and unpleasant.

Eye issues. Many rosacea patients have dry, itchy, and swollen eyes and lids. This is referred to as ocular rosacea. Eye symptoms may occur before, after, or in combination with skin symptoms.

The nose has enlarged. Rosacea may cause the nose's skin to thicken over time, making it seem larger. This disorder is sometimes known as rhinophyma. It happens more often in males than in women.

When to see the doctor.
If you have ongoing facial or ocular issues, see a healthcare expert for diagnosis and treatment plan. Dermatologists are an alternative word for skin care professionals.

Causes
The etiology of rosacea is unknown. It might be related to inheritance, an overactive immune system, or circumstances in your everyday life. Rosacea is not caused by poor hygiene, and you cannot get it from others.

Flare-ups may be caused by:
Sun or breeze.
Hot beverages.
Spicy food.
Alcohol.
Extremely high and low temperatures.
Emotional strain.
Exercise.
Some blood pressure medications are dilation agents.
Various cosmetic, skin, and hair-care items.

Risk Factors:
Anyone may develop rosacea. You might be more prone to develop it if:

I have sun sensitive skin.
   Aged 30 to 50 years.
   Have a history of smoking.
   I have a family member with rosacea.

What Causes Rosacea?

Although the cause of rosacea is unclear, researchers have disco ered key components of the illness, which might lead to substanti breakthroughs in therapy. A recent research found that face redne is most likely the beginning of an inflammatory process caused by combination of neurovascular dysregulation and the innate immur system. The NRS has supported groundbreaking research on th involvement of the innate immune system in rosacea, including th finding of anomalies in critical microbiological components known cathelicidins. An additional study has recently shown that a significai increase in mast cells, which are found at the junction of the neurologic and circulatory systems, is a common connection between all mai symptoms of the illness.

Aside from neurovascular and immune system components, a tiny mit called Demodex folliculorum has been identified as a potential cause c rosacea. This mite is often found on human skin, however, it has bee proven to be substantially more prevalent in the face skin of rosace sufferers. Researchers have also identified two genetic variations in th human genome that may be linked to the illness.

Other recent research has shown links between rosacea and an increase risk of an increasing range of potentially dangerous systemic disorder indicating that rosacea is the result of systemic inflammation. Althoug no causative relationships have been shown, they include cardiovascula sease, gastrointestinal illness, neurological and immunological issues, and various malignancies.

ow is Rosacea treated?

Because the indications and symptoms of rosacea differ, a physician must personalize therapy to each patient's specific needs. Learn more about when to see a doctor.

he disorder's numerous indications and symptoms may be treated with a variety of oral and topical treatments. Physicians may recommend medical treatment, particularly to reduce redness. Bumps and pimples are often treated with oral and topical medications to relieve the symptoms quickly, followed by long-term usage of an anti-inflammatory medication to sustain remission. Rosacea-specific medications are now available in a variety of formulations that may be tailored to the particular patient.

When necessary, lasers, powerful pulsed light sources, or other medical and surgical technologies may be utilized to eliminate visible blood vessels or rectify nasal abnormalities. Ocular rosacea may be treated with anti-inflammatory medicines and other therapies, however, an eye doctor's advice may be required. Rosacea Treatment Photographs offer photos of treatment outcomes.

Skin Care

Patients should consult with their doctors to verify that their skincare routine is appropriate for their rosacea. A mild skin-care program may also assist with rosacea. Patients should wash their faces with a gentle, non-abrasive cleanser, rinse with lukewarm water, and pat dry with a thick cotton towel. Don't pull, tug, or use a scratchy washcloth.

Patients may use non-irritating skin-care products as required, and the should protect their skin from the sun with sunscreen with UVA/UV protection and an SPF of 30 or higher. There are mild or pediatri formulations available for sensitive skin; also, check for non-chemica (mineral) sunscreens with zinc or titanium dioxide. Rosacea sufferei should avoid using skincare products that sting, burn, or produc further redness.

Cosmetics may be used to disguise Rosacea symptoms. To reduc redness, use green makeup or a green-tinted foundation. This may b followed with a skin-tone foundation in natural yellow tones, avoidin; pink and orange shades.

Lifestyle Management
  In addition to long-term medical treatment, rosacea patients ma enhance their odds of remaining in remission by identifying and ad dressing lifestyle and environmental variables that are often associated with flushing and can cause flare-ups or worsen their specific symptom: However, identifying these characteristics is a one-of-a-kind approach since what triggers a flare-up in one individual may not have ar influence on another.

Rosacea sufferers should maintain a record of their daily activities or events and link them to any flare-ups they may have. NRS members may get a Rosacea Diary booklet and other resources for free. Join the NRS now!

Chapter 2

Have you recently been diagnosed with rosacea?
Eight Things You Should Know.

If you've been diagnosed with rosacea, there are numerous steps you may take to relieve symptoms and prevent flare-ups.

A doctor is chatting to a patient.

Were you just diagnosed with Rosacea? If this is the case, you may be wondering what measures to take next. Here are eight pieces of advice that doctors provide their rosacea patients to help them manage the condition and feel more at ease.

1. Pay attention to your eyes. If you don't do anything else, do this! Keep a watch out for signs of irritation or redness in the eyes. If you encounter irritation or other eye problems, call your dermatologist or eye expert right away.

This is noteworthy since more than half of people with rosacea have an eye problem at some point. Treating rosacea-related eye disorders might help you prevent vision problems.

2. Find out what causes your rosacea. Frequent situations, such as being

overheated or stressed, may trigger rosacea to flare. The word "trigge[r]" refers to anything that produces rosacea flare-ups.

While there are various rosacea triggers, what causes one person['s] rosacea may not affect you. It is crucial to understand what is causin[g] your rosacea. Avoiding your triggers might help you avoid flare-ups.

Here's a step-by-step strategy for recognizing your triggers. Trigger[s] may be causing your rosacea flare-ups.

3. Be cautious with your skin. Rosacea may make your skin ver[y] sensitive. If you wash your face with a washcloth, use fragranced o[r] astringent skin care products, or go outdoors without sunscreen, you[r] skin may feel uncomfortable.

You may learn how to care for your rosacea-prone skin by reading th[e] 6 rosacea skin care tips that professionals provide their patients.

4. Protect your skin from the sun. Even a few minutes in the sun ma[y] cause your rosacea to flare. Avoiding sun exposure may help preven[t] these flare-ups.

5. Choose your cosmetics prudently. Cosmetics may worsen rosacea[.] You may discover how to choose rosacea-friendly cosmetics at How to Prevent Rosacea Flare-ups. Scroll down to "Use Rosacea-Friendly Makeup."

6. Understand that flare-ups may happen and are frequently unexpected[.] Even if you treat your rosacea and avoid your triggers, it may flare unexpectedly.

lare-up is more manageable if you stay calm (stress may be a cause)
d adhere to your dermatologist's treatment suggestions.

To cure rosacea, see a board-certified dermatologist. Treating rosacea
y prevent it from deteriorating. Treatment may also help to relieve a
re-up.

board-certified dermatologist can provide specialized therapy for
sacea. When a dermatologist is board-certified, you will see the letters
AD after their name.

Make a list of questions to ask during your next dermatological
pointment. Between sessions, rosacea-related questions may emerge.
they do, write them down so you may ask them at your next
rmatologist appointment.

he more expert help you seek, the better you will be able to control
ur rosacea.

board-certified dermatologist is an expert in rosacea.
Rosacea is among the most common dermatological illnesses.

board-certified dermatologist is a professional who has received
xtensive training in the diagnosis and treatment of rosacea.

oard-certified dermatologists are also the scientists who conduct the
ast bulk of the research that helps us learn more about this problem.

iscover a board-certified dermatologist.

DO YOU NEED TO TREAT ROSACEA?

Rosacea is a prevalent skin ailment that may damage the eyes.

The guy has rosacea around his nose and eyes.

Rosacea afflicted both his eyes and skin. Treatment may help to relie
the rosacea on this man's face and eyes.

When rosacea affects your eyes, therapy is critical. Otherwise, yo
may have vision difficulties. Your eyesight may get obscured. If you ha
severe rosacea in your eyes, you may lose your vision. Early detectic
and treatment of eye issues may help avoid them.

Is rosacea affecting your eyes?

More than half of people with rosacea have eye difficulties at son
time. If you've been diagnosed with rosacea, you need to take speci
care of your eyes. You're looking for:

Swollen and red eyes (the most prevalent symptom).

Red, bloodshot eyes.

Redness and swelling around the eyes.

Crusty lids and lashes.

Tears (or dried eyes)

Feeling like there's something in your eye.

Burning

ching

nsitive to light.

osacea may cause eyesight difficulties before it manifests on the face. When this occurs, your face will not get red or show any other signs. You will experience one or more of the eye disorders mentioned above.

Consult a dermatologist.
If you suspect rosacea is hurting your eyes, schedule an appointment with a dermatologist straight soon.

A woman meets with a doctor.
As previously stated, addressing rosacea-related eye problems may save you from developing vision issues.

Treating eye diseases might also help you avoid a dangerous eye infection. Treatment may also help keep your eyes from feeling dry and gritty.

Treatment may also aid in the removal of crusts on your eyelids and lashes, as well as puffiness around the eyes.

Benefits of Rosacea Treatment for the Skin
When you have rosacea on your skin, therapy might make you feel better. Treatments for your skin may include:

Prevent Rosacea from worsening.

Make you more comfortable.

Increase your self-esteem and quality of life.

Rosacea might worsen if your skin is not treated. Continuous flushing, for example, might leave your face permanently red. Spider veins may develop on the cheekbones. Some individuals get acne-like outbreaks.

These disorders may be avoided with proper skin care.

Treatment for rosacea might also benefit your mental health. Numerous studies have shown that chronic redness, acne-like outbreaks, and other rosacea symptoms may impair one's self-esteem. People often report pain with their skin. Some individuals claim to avoid social situations as much as possible because they are embarrassed.

When rosacea persists for many years, some individuals experience despair, anxiety, or both. Researchers have repeatedly noticed that when rosacea diminishes, so do these symptoms.

Are you worried that your rosacea isn't severe enough to treat?
  People may be reluctant to see a dermatologist until their rosacea becomes severe. Dermatologists recommend that you schedule an appointment well in advance.

The sooner you begin treatment, the simpler it is to control rosacea.

Chapter 3

How to Avoid Rosacea Flare-Ups.

Rosacea is a common skin ailment that causes redness around the nose and cheeks. In addition to seeing a board-certified dermatologist for a correct diagnosis and treatment, people may help manage their disease and keep it from worsening by recognizing and avoiding the triggers that cause their rosacea to flare.

To reduce flare-ups, patients should identify and eliminate aggravating factors for their rosacea.

Think about sun protection.
Even a few minutes of sunshine on rosacea-prone skin may cause uncontrolled flushing and redness. Dermatologists urge that everyone with rosacea

Every day, use a moderate broad-spectrum sunscreen with an SPF of 30 or higher. It is unlikely that a fragrance-free sunscreen containing zinc oxide, titanium dioxide, or both would irritate sensitive skin.

Wear a wide-brimmed hat while spending the day outside.

Stay away from the noon sun.

Seek shade.

Reduce stress.
   If stress causes your rosacea to flare, you may learn how to control it so that it doesn't create another flare-up. Here are some ideas:

Determine a stress-relieving activity and do it on a regular basis. Tai chi, meditation, and joining a rosacea support group are all popular ways to relieve stress.

Do something you like every day.

In a tense situation, take a deep breath, hold it, and then release it gently.

Avoid overheating.
   Dermatologists urge planning ahead of time to avoid heat-related flare-ups.

You can do various things:

Take warm baths and showers instead of hot ones.

Dress in layers so you can remove them if you become too hot.

Feeling overheated? Place a cool, damp towel over your neck. Drink a refreshing drink. Keep cool by using a fan or air conditioning.

far enough away from fireplaces, heaters, and other heat sources to prevent feeling hot.

think hot drinks.
According to studies, hot drinks cause some people's rosacea to flare.

this describes you, a few tweaks may enable you to enjoy drinks that most people drink hot.

y these ideas:

rink iced coffee or tea.

et the liquid cool until it is warm or lukewarm.

xamine the repercussions of alcohol use.
When it comes to alcohol-related flare-ups, red wine may be the leading cause. You may be able to decrease alcohol-induced flares.

rink white wine instead of red.

dd soda or lemonade to white wine, beer, and other alcoholic drinks to reduce the alcohol content.

imit your alcohol consumption to one or two drinks, followed by a big glass of cool water.

t is also recommended to avoid alcohol.

Reduce the frequency of spicy meals.

If spicy foods cause redness in your face, you may be able to enj your favorites by

Attempting a milder rendition. Rather of eating spicy wings that ma you sweat, go for moderate wings. Choose a moderate salsa over a spi one.

If your rosacea is still active, avoid consuming spicy foods.

Carefully choose skin and hair care products.

Do certain skin or hair care products cause your face to burn, stir or itch? Do any of these products make your face dry and scaly? The are signals that they are irritating your skin, which might worsen yo rosacea symptoms.

Here's how to prevent flare-ups:

Consult a physician for a rosacea skin care regimen and produ recommendations.

Avoid using astringents and toners.

Examine the ingredients in all of your skin and hair care product and avoid those that include typical rosacea triggers such as mentho camphor, or sodium lauryl sulfate.

The last component is often found in shampoo and toothpaste. If yo wish to use a product on your face, avoid those with sodium laury sulfate.

pply rosacea-friendly makeup.
If makeup affects your rosacea, you may still be able to use it.

ermatologists recommend:

efore wearing makeup, moisturize your skin with a gentle, fragrance-ee emollient.

sing a lightweight, liquid-based foundation that spreads easily and an be set with powder.

ou want to avoid:

Waterproof makeup

Heavy foundations that don't distribute well and need makeup removal.

Check your medications.
If you believe a medication is causing your rosacea to flare, do not stop using it.

First, ask the doctor who provided the medication whether it is causing your rosacea.

Some medications used to treat rosacea may exacerbate it.

High blood pressure.

Various forms of cardiovascular diseases

Anxiety

Migraines

Glaucoma

Vitamin B3 may also cause Rosacea flare-ups.

whether the drug (or vitamin) is making your face red, ask whether yo
may take another one.

Protect your face from the wind and cold.
   Windburn is prevalent in rosacea-prone skin. Windburn ma
aggravate rosacea, particularly in the winter. Colds may also caus
rosacea.

The following measures may help to decrease flares caused by wind an
cold.

Cover your face with a scarf (up to just below your eyes). Silk and acryli
blend beautifully. Avoid placing wool or other rough-feeling fibers nea
your face, since they may cause a flare-up.

Every day, use rosacea-friendly sunscreen (see "Think sun protection"
and an emollient.

Limit your time outside.

Follow your rosacea treatment plan.

Maintain your composure during exercise.

Anything that elevates your body temperature, including exercise, might cause rosacea. You can still exercise.

There are several strategies to exercise without a flare-up:

Reduce the intensity. You may still benefit from a low- to moderate-intensity workout.

Exercising where it's cool. In the summer, choose an air-conditioned gym or a shaded route during the coolest hours of the day.

Try exercising in water. Swimming in cold water or practicing aqua aerobics may help prevent flares.

Keep stuff around to help you relax. A cold-water-soaked towel, a bottle of cold water, or ice cubes may all help you chill down.

Treat your Rosacea.
Many individuals may avoid rosacea flares by managing their symptoms and avoiding triggers.

A dermatologist can devise a treatment plan to help you manage your signs and symptoms.

Chapter 4

7 ROSACEA SKIN CARE TIPS FROM DERMATOLOGISTS

How To Care For Your Rosacea

An adequate rosacea skincare routine may make you feel more at ease while managing your symptoms. Board certified dermatologists propose the following suggestions.

Rosacea often causes the skin to become sensitive and irritated, therefore proper skin care is critical for controlling the ailment. Proper skin care may include:

Make your skin more comfortable.

Reduce rosacea flare-ups.

Improve the effectiveness of your treatment.

Experts prescribe the following to help you develop a rosacea skin care regimen:

Select rosacea-friendly skincare products. Many skincare and cosmetic items may irritate rosacea sufferers' skin. To reduce the likelihood of using a product that may irritate your skin, experts recommend that you avoid the following ingredients:

Alcohol
Camphor Fragrance
Glycolic acid
Lactic acid
Shampoos and toothpaste often include menthol and sodium lauryl sulfate.
Urea
Go fragrance-free.
Choose fragrance-free (rather than unscented) products to reduce the risk of skin irritation.

To reduce inflammation, it is also advised that:

Choose products that indicate they are gentle on sensitive skin and non-comedogenic (will not clog pores).
Choose a cream instead of a lotion or gel.
Never use an astringent or toner.

Before applying skincare or cosmetics to your face, try them first. Do you feel that everything you apply to your face stings? Testing may help you find products that do not irritate your skin.

You may test goods at home by following these board-certified dermatologists' recommendations on How to Test Skin Care goods.

1. Wash your face twice a day, gently. Cleaning helps to remove oil and

filth, which may cause irritation.

Dermatologists recommend that you clean your skin without irritati
it more.

Select a mild, rosacea-friendly cleanser (not soap).
   Use your fingertips to gently apply the cleaner in a circular motio
   Rinse the cleanser with warm water, using just your fingertips. Y
want to be delicate yet completely remove your cleanser. If any of t
cleanser stays on your skin, it might create irritation.
   Gently wipe your face with a clean cotton cloth.
   Clean your face.
   Cleaning when you get up and before bed eliminates oil and debr
that may irritate your skin.

4. Moisturize after cleaning. Apply your rosacea medication first. The
use a rosacea-friendly moisturizer.

Whether rosacea creates dry or oily skin, moisturizer is essenti
Moisturizing keeps your skin hydrated by retaining water. Moisturizir
also replaces essential lipids in your skin. These changes may mak
your skin less irritating and more comfortable.

According to research, utilizing a rosacea-friendly moisturizer c
barrier repair cream may improve your treatment results.

In one small experiment, people applied rosacea medicine (metronid
zole gel) to their faces twice a day. They used a mild, non-irritatin
hydrating moisturizer to one side of their face twice daily.

ter 15 days, the moisturized side of their face showed less dryness, eeling, and roughness. It also felt more comfortable. Other studies owed similar findings.

pply moisturizer on dry skin.

After washing your face, allow it to dry. Applying moisturizer to dry in minimizes the risk of burning or stinging.

Moisturize your face to protect your skin from the sun all year. The n may worsen rosacea at any time of the year. This is one of the most ommon causes of rosacea flare-ups, and it affects people with all skin nes.

ermatologists recommend the following strategies for reducing sun-duced rosacea flare-ups:

eek shade whenever possible.

Wear sun-protective clothing, including a wide-brimmed hat and JV-blocking sunglasses.

Apply a broad-spectrum sunscreen with an SPF of 30 or higher that s also water resistant. Apply sunscreen to any exposed skin. Even on loudy days, sunscreen is essential.

If a sunscreen affects your skin, choose one that contains:

Zinc oxide, titanium dioxide, or both (sometimes called mineral unscreen).

Silicone is also known as dimethicone, cyclomethicone, or cyclome-hicone.

No fragrance (the label may state "fragrance-free," but if it reads 'unscented" choose another sunscreen)

How to Choose Rosacea-Friendly Sunscreen and Avoid a White Cast.

Certain mineral sunscreens leave a white cast, especially on dark skin tones. To avoid this, doctors recommend using a micronized mineral sunscreen or a tinted mineral sunscreen.

6. Be cautious with your skin. Anything that irritates your skin may cause rosacea flares. To prevent this:

Instead of a washcloth or facial sponge, use your fingers to gently wash and rinse your face.
    Avoid scraping, scouring, or massaging rosacea-prone skin.
    If you exfoliate your skin, stop.

7. Makeup may be applied as desired. A yellow-tinted concealer may cover up discoloration on skin tones ranging from light to dark. A green-tinted concealer may help disguise redness. Keep in mind that some cosmetics may irritate your fragile skin. That is why doctors often recommend water-based or powder cosmetics since they are less prone to irritate your skin.

Including these tactics in your skincare routine will allow you to properly care for your rosacea-prone skin.

If you are having trouble locating sensitive skincare or cosmetics, ask your physician for ideas.

Chapter 5

Rosacea flare-ups: What causes them and how can they be managed?

osacea is a chronic inflammatory condition characterized by visible and swollen blood vessels on the face, as well as redness and tiny pus-filled pimples. It might be triggered by a range of meals, stress, or other circumstances. Techniques for keeping the face hydrated may aid with this.

According to study, around 5.46% of people worldwide have rosacea. However, healthcare providers may misdiagnose the symptoms as acne or psoriasis.

People with rosacea may experience both remission and flare-ups, which are times of heightened symptoms. Patients often pinpoint particular conditions that trigger flare-ups. Certain foods, heat, weather, stress, and medications are all possible reasons.

Although rosacea is painful and incurable, there are numerous therapies available to help patients control their flare-ups.

This page discusses rosacea flare-ups, including causes, treatment options, and prevention.

What causes rosacea flare-ups?

Rosacea sufferers have very sensitive skin, so a variety of circumstances may provoke flare-ups. For example, sun exposure may promote long-term skin redness and flushing. Skin care products may irritate, burn, and itch.

Doctors use the word "trigger" to describe the variables that produce rosacea flare-ups. Triggers varied amongst persons, although they often included:

Some of the delights accessible include dairy products, liver, citrus fruits, vinegar, chocolate, soy sauce, beans, and spicy dishes.

Alcoholic beverages include red wine, beer, and spirits, as well as heated liquids such as tea and coffee.

Tension and worry are two emotions.

Cosmetics include skin and hair care goods including hairspray, witch hazel, acetone, and alcohol.

Hot baths, saunas, and warm environments are all examples of heat therapies.

Weather: sun, cold, humidity, and strong winds.

Physical exertion includes lifting and loading heavy items, as well as other strenuous tasks.

There are two sorts of medications: topical steroids and vasodilators.

Menopause, chronic cough, and caffeine withdrawal syndrome are instances of medical conditions.

How to Reduce Rosacea Flare-ups

Those who avoid triggers may notice that their rosacea flares up less often.

The suggestions below may also be useful:

A mild, fragrance-free moisturizer might help to relax the skin.
Using a humidifier may help keep dry air from removing moisture from your skin.
Drink lots of water to stay hydrated and keep your skin from drying.
Wrap a cold water-soaked cloth over your neck.
Engage in stress-relieving hobbies like yoga and meditation.

How long does a flare-up last?

The duration of a rosacea flare-up varies from person to person, making it hard to predict. However, anecdotal data shows that it might range from days to months.

Rosacea is a chronic disorder that alternates between remission and relapses, often known as flare-ups. A retrospective study of 48 persons with rosacea found that 52% had active rosacea for an average of 13 years. The remaining 48% had rosacea cured after an average of 9 years.

According to research, those who continue to their rosacea treatments over time are less likely to have flare-ups.

Preventing flare-ups.

People may help prevent rosacea flare-ups by identifying and avoidi
their causes. Keeping note of what they eat and drink, what activit:
they do, where they travel, and their rosacea symptoms may helr
person identify the triggers for flare-ups.

The following tips may also help people avoid rosacea flare-ups:

Sun protection: Apply a moderate broad-spectrum sunscreen wi
an SPF of 30 or higher every day. Choose fragrance-free sunscree
with zinc oxide, titanium dioxide, or both, since they are less irritatir
People should wear broad-brimmed hats and avoid direct sunlight.

Reduce stress: Tai chi and meditation are two strategies that m:
help people reduce stress. In addition, stress management breathir
techniques might be useful in stressful circumstances.

To avoid overheating, wear in layers, take warm or cold bat]
and showers, and stay away from direct heat sources like fires. A
conditioning, fans, and cold beverages may all help individuals kee
cool.

Choose cold beverages over hot tea or coffee.

Rethink your beverage selections. Drink white wine instead of re
and mix alcoholic drinks with soda or lemonade.

Choose appropriate cosmetics: Your dermatologist may offer rosace
friendly skin care products. Avoid astringents, toners, and product
containing menthol, camphor, or sodium laurel sulfate.

Check medications: If a person suspects that a medicine is causing
rosacea flare, they should see their doctor about alternatives. Howeve
it is critical not to discontinue the drug without first treating th
problem.

Treatment

Doctors do not have a treatment for rosacea, however the following approaches may help alleviate symptoms:

Oral antibiotics

Doctors often recommend tetracycline antibiotics, such as doxycline and minocycline, for their anti-inflammatory qualities and ability to kill bacteria on the skin. A course typically lasts 6 to 12 weeks, depending on the individual's symptoms. Individuals may need additional courses from time to time.

Topical medications.

Metronidazole cream or gel may be used alone or alongside oral antibiotics. To reduce swelling and redness, doctors may give azelaic acid, brimonidine gel, sulfacetamide sodium, sulfacetamide sulfur, or topical ivermectin.

After months of drug use, a person's rosacea symptoms may improve.

Doctors may provide the following treatments for rosacea.

Lasers and strong pulsed light treatment are used to eliminate enlarged blood vessels.

Electrocautery uses electricity to remove damaged blood vessels, while dermabrasion removes the top layer of the skin.

Rosacea is an inflammatory skin disorder characterized by swollen blood vessels and face redness.

People with rosacea often have periods of no symptoms followed by flare-ups. Food, medicine, heat, and stress are common reasons.

People may attempt to control flare-ups by identifying and avoiding their triggers. Furthermore, keeping the skin hydrated and cold during a flare-up may assist in alleviating symptoms.

People who utilize long-term rosacea therapies are less likely to have severe flare-ups.

What are the similarities and differences between rosacea and acne.

Rosacea and acne are skin conditions that may affect the face. Acne and rosacea patients may have red, inflamed skin, pimples, or sensitive skin.

Rosacea, on the other hand, is a distinct condition with its own set of symptoms.

This chapter looks at the similarities and differences between rosacea and acne, as well as how to treat each.

Overview

Another name for rosacea is "acne rosacea." Regardless, it is a distinct disorder from acne vulgaris, sometimes known as "acne."

It may be difficult to differentiate between rosacea and acne. Treatments, however, differ from person to person, hence a thorough diagnosis is vital for guaranteeing early and adequate treatment.

It is conceivable to be in both circumstances simultaneously.

There are various kinds of rosacea, including:

Erythematotelangiectatic Rosacea.
People with this kind of rosacea may experience:

Symptoms may include flushing of the face, redness around the nose and cheeks, and visible blood vessels.
Papulopustular Rosacea.
Individuals with this kind of rosacea have:

Painful acne-like breakouts with whiteheads.
Common symptoms include swelling and red bumps.
Ocular rosacea.
This kind of rosacea affects the eyes. People with ocular rosacea may experience:

Watery eyes.
Bloodshot eyes.
Symptoms may include stinging and weird physical sensation.
Burning feeling and blurred vision.
sensitive to light.
Phymatous Rosacea
This unusual kind of rosacea primarily affects males. Patients with phymatous rosacea could have:

Symptoms may include thickened skin on the nose, chin, forehead, cheeks, or ears, as well as irregular lumps in certain locations.
Bulbous nose.

What is acne?
Acne vulgaris is the most widespread chronic skin disorder in the United States, affecting about 50 million persons yearly.

It produces skin lesions, or pimples, on the face, chest, and upper back.

The lesions might be whiteheads, blackheads, inflammatory papules, nodules, pustules, or cysts.

Similarities and Differences

The table below compares and contrasts rosacea with acne, according to the American Academy of Dermatology (AAD).

	Rosacea	Acne
Age of onset	It typically occurs in those older than 30 years of age, but it can start earlier or later in some people.	Teenagers and preteens are most likely to get acne, although it can affect people of any age.
Who it impacts	Fair-skinned people are most likely to develop rosacea, but people of all races and colors can develop it.	People of all races and colors can develop acne.
Location	The most common places to develop rosacea are the face and eyes. However, the redness may extend to a person's chest, neck, scalp, or upper back.	Acne typically develops on the face, jawline, chest, neck, upper back, and shoulders.
Redness or inflammation	Yes, this can come and go or be permanent and typically appears on the cheeks, forehead, nose, or chin area.	Yes, the skin may be red or inflamed around the breakouts only.
Breakouts	Pimple-like breakouts may occur in some cases.	Whiteheads, blackheads, pimples, or painful cysts or nodules may appear.
Blackheads	No	Yes
Oily skin	No	Yes, usually on the "T-zone" area of the forehead, nose, and chin.
Large pores	Yes	Yes
Texture	The skin may be thick or bumpy, especially with phymatous rosacea.	The skin may be bumpy due to scarring or active blemishes.
Eye problems	If a person experiences ocular rosacea, they may have red or swollen eyelids, bloodshot eyes, and discomfort in the eyes.	No
Visible blood vessels	Yes	No
Sensitive skin	Burning, stinging, or itching may occur due to skin care products or makeup.	Sometimes

Causes

Both acne and rosacea may have hereditary roots because having a family member with either condition can increase one's own risk.

Rosacea might be brought on by demodex mites. While all skin has these mites, those with rosacea often have larger concentrations of them.

The AAD claims that this idea is flawed because many people who not have rosacea also have a high concentration of Demodex mites their skin.

Acne can be brought on by abnormal cell clumping in the follic] excessive sebum production, or bacteria on the skin.

Recognition

People should see a dermatologist in order to determine the natu of their skin issue.

The symptoms may also be suggestive of another condition complete such as contact dermatitis or perioral dermatitis.

Dermatologists can run tests to rule out other conditions that cou. mimic rosacea or acne.

A doctor can diagnose a condition based on a patient's medical histor appearance of the skin and eyes, and other variables. Trusted Source

Treatment for Rosacea

Treatment for rosacea focuses on symptom management, stoppin the disease's progression or repercussions, and improving the qualit of life for individuals who have it, as there is currently no known cur for the condition.

There are several different ways to treat rosacea, including Truste Sources:

topical gels, creams, and ointments containing antibiotics

Topical antiparasitics to reduce the amount of Demodex mites on the skin, topical vasoconstrictors to minimize the appearance of blood vessels, and oral antibiotics

Retinoids are lubricating drops for the eyes that may be helpful in reducing the size and appearance of blood vessels using laser and light therapy.

People should also avoid doing anything that they know could exacerbate their disease.

Applying sunscreen outside and avoiding triggers such as: are two ways to prevent this.

Hot drinks with alcohol

high temps, severe gusts, and hot food with caffeine

Acne treatments

As with rosacea, the objectives of acne treatment Source are to block the emergence of new symptoms and relieve existing ones.

Some therapies focus on the underlying causes of acne.

Among these therapies are topical medicines such as:

drugs to remove microorganisms

Benzoyl peroxide to destroy microorganisms

Resorcinol, sulfur, or salicylic acid can be used to eliminate blackheads and whiteheads.

Retinoids for the treatment of inflammation and lesions

Other therapies might be:

retinoids, chemical peels, oral antibiotics, laser and light therapy

Furthermore, people ought to avoid anything that can irritate the acne.

It is best to refrain from pinching, caressing, rubbing, or picking at faults as these behaviors may cause scarring.

Summary: Despite their apparent similarities, acne vulgaris and acne rosacea are two separate forms of skin diseases.

Dermatologists can distinguish between the two conditions based only on a patient's skin, even though there are differences between the two.

Skin outbreaks resulting in blackheads and whiteheads can be caused by anxiety. Rosacea can result in pimples but does not produce blackheads.

Rosacea cannot coexist with acne, but oily skin can. Two more rosacea side effects include visible blood vessels and eye issues.

For either illness, there is no treatment. As such, the goals of treatment for both are to reduce symptoms and try to stop new ones from arising.

II

Part Two

Natural Treatments for Rosacea

In this part you will discover various natural remedies for Rosacea, each remedies options you in the following chapters may be repeated,fear not they all have different ingredients and prescriptions

Chapter 6

guide to natural therapies for Rosacea

Certain natural remedies seem to alleviate rosacea symptoms.

Rosacea is an inflammatory condition marked by a crimson or discolored rash on the cheeks and nose, which may also develop on the forehead, chin, and eyes.

Rosacea has no cure. However, there are various treatment choices. Some treatments are accessible in nature and may be performed at home.

This chapter outlines some of the natural therapies for rosacea.

Natural cures for Rosacea.
Nancybelle Gonzaga Villarroya/Getty Images.
Before trying any natural or alternative rosacea treatments, consumers should contact with a healthcare professional. They should

clarify whatever medications they are presently taking to verify th
there are no adverse reactions to any natural or herbal therapies.

It is also crucial to do a patch test with any new products, since so
people may have adverse reactions.

Aloe vera

Aloe vera gel, found on the inside of the plant's long, pointed leav
is an emollient and moisturizer that may help treat rosacea. This is d
in part to the belief that aloe vera has anti-inflammatory properties.
also moisturizes the skin and may help reduce redness.

The gel formed from the leaves may be applied directly to the skin.
also appears in a number of skincare products.

Burdock

Burdock is a root that has long been used in traditional treatments
Europe, North America, and Asia. It is said to improve blood circulatio
to the skin, resulting in increased skin brightness and evenness.

It has anti-inflammatory and antibacterial properties, as well as antio
idant activity. These characteristics may be effective in treating th
symptoms of skin illnesses like rosacea.

Burdock may be found in several forms, such as:

Fresh roots
   Burdock Tea.
   Burdock Root Dry Powder
   Burdock oil or extracts.

Chamomile

Chamomile contains antiinflammatory properties. As a consequence, is often utilized in rosacea treatments.

may be used as an essential oil when diluted, or cooled tea can be applied directly to the skin via soaking compresses.

Coconut oil.

Coconut oil is an effective moisturizer. There has been no recent study on the efficacy of coconut oil for rosacea. However, researchTrusted Source shows that it has anti-inflammatory, antioxidant, and moisturizing effects. These benefits may help to relieve the inflamed skin associated with rosacea.

Coconut oil works best when applied directly to wet or moist skin, such as immediately after a shower. It may also be used as a carrier oil to dilute essential oils for topical use.

Comfrey

Comfrey is a plant that contains allantoins. This is a substance that may help with skin reactions.

A 2017 study on a product containing allantoin found that it alleviated symptoms with little to no side effects. It also seems to help reduce skin redness.

This is commercially available in products that list comfrey or allantoin as ingredients.

Feverfew

Feverfew, another plant from the chamomile family, is often used to treat rosacea. It has antioxidant and anti-inflammatory properties.

Feverfew also shields the skin from UV rays and other environmenta variables that might cause skin damage, such as heat, inflammation, an smoking.

This is commercially available in numerous products advertised to trea a range of ailments. It is recommended that you use a parthenolide-fre product since parthenolide might cause skin irritation.

Green tea

Green tea has significant quantities of antioxidants. Antioxidants hel to reduce inflammation in the body, especially in the skin. According to a 2021 study, green tea may be an effective treatment for a numbe of skin problems. Rosacea may be among them.

Green tea is marketed as both a herbal beverage and an oral supplement A person may take tea for systemic benefits. They may also apply coolec green tea to their skin using a moist cloth.

Lavender essential oil

Many essential oils may assist with skin conditions like rosacea Lavender is a common natural treatment for rosacea. It's also a commonly used essential oil.

A few drops of lavender oil may be mixed with another oil, such as coconut oil, or blended into any moisturizer. Essential oils should never be swallowed and must always be diluted before use on the skin

Although studies show that essential oils may have health benefits, it is important to highlight that the Food and Drug Administration (FDA) does not monitor or oversee their purity or quality.

Before using essential oils, speak with a healthcare professional and research the quality of the products supplied by a certain firm. Before experimenting with a new essential oil, always do a patch test.

Niacinamide

Niacinamide is a B vitamin found in food. It may reduce some of the redness associated with rosacea. It has been shown to have anti-inflammatory properties and to protect the skin from environmental stressors and aging.

Niacinamide is included in creams and lotions used to treat inflammatory skin conditions. In this form, it may help to prevent and cure rosacea-related flushing.

Oatmeal

Oatmeal is a popular and efficient treatment for skin irritation because it improves the skin's capacity to retain moisture. According to study from 2018Trusted Source, oatmeal has anti-inflammatory and antioxidant properties. This might help to lessen the look of rosacea indirectly.

Many irritated or inflamed skin care solutions use oats. It may also be combined with water and used directly to the skin, or added to a bath to soak.

Raw honey.

Raw honey may help to reduce the redness and inflammation caused

by rosacea. Honey helps the skin maintain moisture, which may b
useful for rosacea. A 2015 study found that kanuka honey may hel
cure rosacea.

High-quality raw kanuka or manuka honey may be applied on the ski

Lifestyle Changes to Manage Rosacea
   Lifestyle changes may also assist with rosacea symptoms, especially
they avoid previously identified irritants. Changes may include:

Managing Stress
   Applying sunscreen and wearing sun-protective clothing may hel
limit UV exposure.
   Applying modest skin care products on delicate skin.
   Following a Mediterranean diet.

Rosacea Treatment Options
   Before exploring any potential rosacea treatments, contact with
healthcare specialist. Prescription drugs consist of the following:

Brimonidine may be used topically.
   Azelaic acid.
   Oral Doxycycline (or other oral Tetracyclines)
   Metronidazole may be used topically.
   Topical oxymetazoline.
   ivermectin
   sulfacetamide-sulfur
   Oral isotretinoin (for severe cases that have not responded to earlier
treatments).
   Laser and intense pulsed light treatment
   Summary

There are various natural ways to treat rosacea symptoms. Aloe vera, coconut oil, and lavender are among the alternatives.

Lifestyle changes, like as stress management and sun protection, may also help to lessen the frequency of rosacea flare-ups.

Before using any treatment, whether natural or medical, one should contact with a healthcare professional.

Chapter 7

5 Home Remedies For Rosacea

We are all known that Rosacea is a long-term skin illne characterized by flushing of the face, especially the nos and cheeks, and the development of tiny acne-like pimpl Rosacea is characterized by both remissions and flare-ups along i course. Remissions are periods of time when your rosacea symptom disappear, but flare-ups cause them to recur

Rosacea cannot be cured, but it may be controlled well. You may trea rosacea by following your dermatologist's advice, avoiding aggravatin situations, and sticking to specific skincare guidelines.

Treatments include:

Rosacea treatment methods aim to alleviate or manage the illness. Thes options may be provided in customized combinations for each patien

There are various medical treatments for rosacea, including:

Cleansers/face washes (sulpha, azelaic acid, benzoyl peroxide)
Topical creams (metronidazole, clindamycin, erythromycin)
Antibiotic pills (tetracycline, doxycycline, minocycline)
Isotretinoin tablets (Accutane) are commonly used as a last option after other oral medications fail.
Lasers may remove thicker skin and blood vessels.
Pulsed-light treatments include the use of controlled light to reduce redness and tiny bumps or pimples.
Photodynamic therapy is putting a topical photosensitizer liquid to the skin and activating it with light.
Some acne drugs (tretinoin, adapalene, and tazarotene)
Seek early treatment so that your doctor can build the optimal treatment plan for you after a thorough assessment.

How To Avoid Rosacea Triggers

To maximize the effects of rosacea treatment, avoid the triggers that cause your rosacea to flare. Sun exposure, mental stress, hot and spicy foods, low temperatures, and other factors are all common causes.

You may begin by maintaining a notebook in which you can make daily notes on the foods you consume and the activities you engage in, and then evaluate if these are the triggering factors for your rosacea. As a consequence, you may try to avoid such triggers by doing things like not going out in the midday sun, applying sunscreen while outdoors, doing something you like to reduce stress, and so on.

Wash your face twice a day with a gentle cleanser, being careful not to overdo it.
Apply sunscreen with SPF 50 at least 15 minutes before going

outdoors.

Avoid cleansing your face.

Avoid using cosmetics and hair sprays that include sodium lauryl ethyl sulfate (SLES).

Alcohol and other irritating ingredients (such as menthol or camphor) should be avoided in soaps, moisturizers, and sunscreens.

Apply face moisturizers carefully to prevent the skin from drying out.

What's the greatest home remedy for Rosacea?

There is no home remedy that has been shown to be the best effective for rosacea. Several studies, however, demonstrate that natural treatment may be especially effective in people who are very sensitive to a variety of topical medications. Some of the possible home treatments include:

Apply diluted white vinegar soaks or wash the skin daily or weekly with a solution of one part regular table vinegar and six parts water. Diluting the vinegar is very important.

Apply green tea soaks on your face.

Apply oatmeal, niacinamide, feverfew, licorice, teas, coffeeberry, aloe vera, chamomile, turmeric, and mushroom extracts (which have been reported to alleviate rosacea symptoms).

Massage your face softly in a circular motion, starting in the middle and extending outward to your ears. Before touching the face, make sure your hands are clean and sanitized.

Consider eating an anti-inflammatory diet (like the Mediterranean diet).

Does rosacea fade away?

Rosacea will not disappear completely since there is no cure. However, is does not suggest that it will become worse with time. You may ontrol it by using a number of treatments and preventive measures ainst the causes.

ome kinds of rosacea respond well to long-term treatment with ser, pulse-light treatments, photodynamic therapy, or isotretinoin. lthough they are not considered a "cure," they may give long-term enefits, improve your skin health, and maybe slow or reverse the ourse of the illness.

What happens if rosacea goes untreated?
It is estimated that more than 16 million people in the United States uffer with rosacea, although many go untreated or postpone getting reatment.

acial flushing during early rosacea is short, lasting anywhere from a ew minutes to many hours. If not treated, rosacea may worsen and roduce permanent redness. Rhinophymas are little, knobby pimples hat appear on the nose. The eyes may become red and dry, and in rare nstances, severely impacted. If not treated, the disease may impair ision.

Natural Remedies for Rosacea

Do pink cheeks make you feel less than happy? Rosacea doesn't have to ruin your holiday season. Try these five simple natural remedies…

People suppose you are always embarrassed. However, rosacea sufferers

are aware that the constant pink tint, known as "flushing," is a sympto:
of rosacea, a skin disease that involves inflammation and dilatation
hundreds of tiny blood vessels near the skin's surface. The Nation
Institutes of Health estimates that around 14 million Americans have

Aside from redness, which may intensify over time, symptoms ma
include acne-like pimples, visible blood vessels, facial swelling, a warr
sensation in the face, and dry or red eyes.

While rosacea is assumed to be a vascular disorder characterized b
increased blood flow, the exact causes are uncertain. Sun exposur
extreme heat or cold, mental stress, strenuous exercise, spicy foods, an
alcohol are some of the most common triggers for those affected.

Many individuals get relief with medical treatments such as ora
antibiotics, prescription creams, and laser therapy.

However, natural remedies may also be useful in easing symptom
Here are a few recommendations that could be useful.

1. Try natural anti-inflammatories.

Many herbs may assist in alleviating rosacea flushing.

"Several herbal ingredients found in a variety of beauty product:
can reduce inflammation and soothe the skin," says dermatologist Joe
Schlessinger, M.D., from Omaha, Nebraska.

ere are six herbal plants that top doctors
commend:

vender: This Mediterranean plant has long been used to treat a
nge of skin disorders, including rashes, pimples, and rosacea. When
plied topically, lavender decreases inflammation and constricts facial
ood vessels.

The oil extracted from lavender leaves is marketed as a therapeutic-
ade (purest and safest) essential oil that may be applied directly to the
in.

"If you only had one naturally soothing ingredient in your cleansing
d beauty products, lavender is the best bet," says Carl Thornfeldt,
.D., a board-certified clinical dermatologist in Fruitland, Idaho.

2008 study done at China's University of Science and Technology
und that licorice extract is a potent anti-inflammatory for skin cells.
hat's because licorice root (also known as sweet root or glycyrrhiza
abra) includes coumarins, flavonoids, plant sterols, and glycyrrhizin,
l of which assist in reducing rosacea redness.

According to a 2006 study presented to the American Academy of
ermatology, licorice extract products enhanced results in those who
ad previously received prescription rosacea treatments.

everfew: A 2010 University of Louisville study discovered that using
his herb topically prevents blood from collecting in facial capillaries.
his indicates less tiny red lines during rosacea flare-ups.

Green tea is thought to help fight cancer and heart disease. Re-
archers have now included rosacea on the list of health benefits when
eated topically. It is an anti-inflammatory and antioxidant that lessens
 he skin's susceptibility to UV radiation, so helping to prevent sun-
nduced flare-ups.

A brief 2010 Case Western Reserve University study discovered th
epigallocatechin-3-gallate (EGCG), the principal polyphenol comp
nent of tea, prevented papules and pustules on the faces of rosac
patients.

Oatmeal, a breakfast staple, might also help to relieve itchy and d
skin.

"These same properties, in turn, promote the skin's natural abili
to protect itself from inflammatory attacks like rosacea," added Sc
lessinger.

Oatmeal also acts as a skin protectant and exfoliant.

"Your skin will have a normal healthy glow instead of being flushe
or red," added the dermatologist.

Chamomile: "Chamomile is a popular ingredient because it has mar
active components that reduce inflammation," Thornfeldt says.

A 2005 study published in the Journal of the European Academy
Dermatology and Venereology discovered that chamomile-based lotio
was an effective treatment for moderate rosacea.

To make a chamomile compress at home, steep two tea bags for 3
seconds in warm (not hot or boiling) water. Pat them dry (making sur
not to wring out every last drop of moisture) and check the temperatur
on your wrist to ensure it is not too hot. Apply one bag to each chee
for 10 minutes.

Caution: Some people are sensitive to chamomile, especially if the
are allergic to ragweed, marigolds, or daisies.

2. Read skin-care product labels carefully.

There is a considerable difference between what cosmetic manufac
turers advertise and what is really in the jar.

"There are no [government] guidelines for how much of a natura medy must be in a cleanser or cream," said Schlessinger.

A product's purity and "natural" ingredients may also be problematic. ow can you know whether you're getting the optimum concentration?

"Look for products made with organic versions of these ingredients ensure you're using the highest quality and reducing the chance that nything artificial might trigger a flare," recommends Cecilia Wong, an sthetician and owner of Soie Aroma Spa in Manhattan.

Thornfeldt claims that natural remedies may take up to three weeks dramatically reduce redness and other symptoms, regardless of the omponents employed.

. Eliminate any food allergies.

Your extravagant holiday diet of pies, deviled eggs, and cakes may rigger a flare-up. During an allergic reaction to food, blood vessels ilate or open wide, generating a tidal wave of blood flow to the skin nd causing redness.

"Corn, egg, and wheat allergies are common in people with rosacea," ays Kimberly Wilson, N.M.D., founder of the Innovations Wellness Center in Plano, Texas.

"The easiest way to tell if the flushing symptoms might be caused y dietary allergies is to eliminate these foods for 2-3 weeks and then gradually add them back one at a time, to test for a possible reaction."

. Switch your pillowcases.

Skin oils, filth, and dead skin cells may accumulate on pillows and log pores as you sleep.

"That often results in the bumps and pimples of rosacea, similar to hose seen in acne," Wilson said.

Change your pillowcase every other day to eliminate filth and grease. Sleep on side "A" the first night after putting on a new case. When you wake up, flip the pillow over to side "B" so it is ready for the next night.

Wash your pillows and linens using hypoallergenic laundry soap that has no added colors or odors.

Additionally, replace synthetic pillows with white cotton ones.

Synthetic materials and colors may cause discomfort and inflammation.

5. De-stress.

"Stress can exacerbate rosacea, so it's important to learn to cope with stress constructively to minimize symptoms," says Thornfeldt.

"Often, the stress of feeling self-conscious about your rosacea symptoms will exacerbate them, causing a rosacea flare."

Meditation, yoga, or even taking a few deep breaths may help you calm and cope.

When you're feeling nervous, the National Rosacea Society suggests taking a deep breath to the count of 10 and gradually exhaling while counting to ten. Repeat until you feel relaxed.

Alternatively, close your eyes and imagine a pleasant place, such as a beach, picnic spot, or your patio, while sitting quietly for a few minutes.

The material on www.Lifescript.com (the "Site") is provided only for informational reasons and is not meant to substitute the advice of your doctor or healthcare professional. This information should not be used to diagnose or treat a health problem or sickness, or to prescribe medications. When dealing with any medical condition, always seek the advice of a qualified healthcare professional. The information and representations on this website about dietary supplements have not been evaluated by the Food and Drug Administration and are not intended to diagnose, treat, cure, or prevent any disease. Lifescript offers no recommendations or endorsements for any specific tests, physicians, third-party products, services, opinions, or other content

pressed on the Site.   Relying on any information provided by
ifescript is solely at your own discretion.

6 Natural Remedies for Rosacea

reen tea, raw honey, and aloe vera are natural remedies that can help
:duce redness and discomfort.

you have rosacea, you are aware that flushing and redness can be
ncomfortable. When confronted with an unexpected trigger, you wish
iere was a way to simply tell your skin to chill!

'ortunately, treatments exist to help soothe rosacea-affected skin.
Vhile medical professionals do not fully understand this chronic skin
ondition, there are several therapies that may help and should be
onsidered. Some natural remedies may also help you relax.

)ermatologist Wilma Bergfeld, MD, explains what rosacea is, how to
reat it naturally, and what lifestyle changes can help reduce redness.

f you have severe rosacea, your doctor or dermatologist will prescribe
intihistamines or, in rare cases, surgery or laser treatments. "Most of
hese treatments are still evolving," says Dr. Bergfeld. "But their goal is
o dampen the expansion of the blood vessels."

Iowever, natural therapies and lifestyle changes may help you manage
rour symptoms. It's important to note that these treatments may
iot work for everyone, so consult with a healthcare professional or

dermatologist before attempting any of them.

Here are some known or studied natural remedies for rosacea

Natural Treatment Options for Rosacea

While none of these natural therapies are likely to cure or completely manage rosacea, they may be beneficial, particularly in terms of lowering inflammation and redness.

Aloe vera

Aloe vera is well-known for its ability to soothe sunburns. Similarly, aloe vera's calming qualities may alleviate rosacea-caused skin irritation and inflammation. Try applying pure aloe vera gel (store-bought or cut straight from the plant) to the afflicted regions to see whether it cools and lowers redness.

Green tea

There's a reason you've seen green tea as an ingredient in several skin products: the regular tea you drink in the morning contains anti-inflammatory and antioxidant characteristics that may benefit your skin.

Several studies have looked at the impact of green tea on giving ultraviolet (UV) protection to the skin, so if you have rosacea flare-ups caused by sun exposure, it may be able to help decrease redness and form a protective barrier.

You may use green tea extract in a topical basis or apply green tea bags to your face.

Oatmeal

You've undoubtedly heard that oatmeal masks are a relaxing, natural treatment for your face.

Using it as a mild cleanser or soothing face mask will help reduce rosacea-related discomfort.

Oatmeal's anti-inflammatory qualities may help relax and soothe irritated skin while also reducing redness and irritation.

In addition, oatmeal may work as a mild exfoliator, removing dead skin cells and unclogging pores without causing more irritation, which may improve the overall texture and look of rosacea-affected skin.

To use oatmeal, combine finely ground oats with water to make a paste and apply it to your face for 15 to 20 minutes before washing.

Chamomile

Chamomile tea bags may have a relaxing impact on your skin, much like a cup of chamomile tea may before bed. Several studies have shown that chamomile has moisturizing characteristics that may help alleviate skin irritation. It may help calm and reduce skin inflammation, itching, and pain caused by rosacea.

This may be especially beneficial during rosacea flare-ups when your skin becomes more sensitive and reactive. To relieve rosacea symptoms, use cooled chamomile tea bags or utilize chamomile-based skincare products.

Lavender and Tea Tree essential oils

Essential oils include anti-inflammatory and antibacterial qualities, which may help with rosacea. "Tea tree oil and a few other botanicals are used to dampen the inflammation," says Dr. Bergfeld.

A 2022 research evaluating multiple therapies for rosacea discover
that tea tree oil may help eradicate the tiny mites that trigger rosac
inflammation.

However, since essential oils may be powerful, they must be adequate
diluted before being applied to your face. Before using essential oils
your skin, consult your doctor or a dermatologist.

Raw honey

We are aware of several of honey's health advantages. However, ra
honey may help lessen the redness and irritation associated with rosac
But you don't want to simply take any honey off the grocery store she
go for raw, all-natural honey with no additional additives. Kanuka
manuka honey, in particular, helps to keep the afflicted skin moist.

Lifestyle adjustments may assist with rosacea.

What you put on your skin does not have to be the only facto
influencing your rosacea. Along with attempting natural therapi
and keeping your healthcare physician informed, you may make certai
lifestyle adjustments to help reduce the redness to a minimum.

Here are some lifestyle changes that might be beneficial:

Reduce stress. Stress may trigger Rosacea flare-ups. Stress managemer
activities such as meditation, deep breathing exercises, and yoga ma
help lessen stress and maybe improve symptoms.

Skincare. Use gentle, non-irritating skin care products created partic
ularly for sensitive skin. Avoid using harsh cleansers, exfoliants, an

brasive scrubbing, which may increase rosacea symptoms. Choose fragrance-free, non-comedogenic products. It's also a good idea to keep a regular skin care program and avoid making frequent product changes. Sudden adjustments or considerable experimentation with skincare could irritate your skin and aggravate rosacea symptoms.

Use sun protection. UV radiation may exacerbate flare-ups of rosacea, so protect your skin from the sun. Wear a broad-spectrum sunscreen with an SPF of 30 or higher every day, even on cloudy days. Also, wear hats and seek shade during high sunlight hours. Dr. Bergfeld believes that wearing protective headgear is your best alternative, as some sunscreens may have an adverse influence on rosacea.

Know your triggers. Identify and prevent sources that exacerbate your rosacea symptoms. Spicy foods, hot beverages, alcohol, caffeine, harsh temperatures, wind, and certain skin-care products are all typical causes. Keeping a journal of your flare-ups can help you find particular reasons.

The bottom line
While there is no cure for rosacea, natural therapy and lifestyle changes may help control the symptoms. Remember that your rosacea experience may vary from others, so see a healthcare professional or dermatologist before selecting which treatment options are best for you. You may lessen your symptoms by taking appropriate care, avoiding triggers, and developing a specific approach.

Chapter 8

There are 19 natural treatments for Rosacea.

ensitive skin is prone to irritation and flare-ups, which may progress to chronic skin conditions such as rosacea. Natural remedies offer a fantastic therapeutic effect, lowering redness, inflammation, and other unpleasant symptoms.

This essay looks at nineteen natural rosacea cures that you may start utilizing right now.

Natural rosacea cures.

Can Rosacea be healed naturally?

19 Treatments and Tips

Rosacea is a common inflammatory skin condition that produces flushing or persistent redness in the central face (nose, chin, and cheeks). Other symptoms include burning, stinging, rough or scaly skin, and spider veins. Flare-ups occur in cycles, exacerbated by environmental causes such as prolonged sun exposure or stress.

thorough skincare plan, along with natural skincare products, may sist to soothe and relieve pain. Here are some tried-and-true natural lutions for rosacea.

Aloe Vera.
Aloe vera has soothing, antioxidant, and moisturizing properties that ay help alleviate rosacea symptoms. Its potent blend of vitamins, inerals, and amino acids forms a protective barrier that prevents oisture loss while soothing skin irritations. Aloe vera also has wound-ealing capabilities, which promote cell turnover and repair wounded ssue, providing quick relief.

he gel extracted from this succulent is often used in moisturizers, unscreens, serums, and face masks. That's why we included it in our pecial mask, Vibrant Skin CBD Recovery Mask.

ibrant Skin CBD Recovery Mask is a natural treatment option for osacea.
Shop now:

) Chamomile
This herbal medicine is effective for dry, irritated skin. Its delicate otanical properties hydrate, soothe, and protect injured skin. Its asoconstrictive effects reduce redness and dilated blood vessels, naking it ideal for rosacea patients.

hamomile is an active ingredient in natural skincare products like LASTIN's Soothe and Protect Recovery Balm.

LASTIN Soothe and Protect Recovery Balm is a natural treatment for osacea.

Shop now.

You may also apply diluted chamomile oil directly to your skin o use cooled chamomile tea as a cold compress but only use produc containing natural chamomile extract.

3. Coconut Oil.

Coconut oil includes antioxidants and fatty acids, which aid i minimizing water loss, reducing inflammation, and maintaining th skin's barrier. It also includes a high concentration of lauric acid, whic has strong antibacterial properties and is good for sensitive, dry, o flushed skin.

Osmosis Remedy MD Healing Balm contains coconut oil and othe herbs that soothe sensitive skin, promote skin density, and provid enough hydration. You may also apply small quantities of high-qualit coconut oil or use it as a carrier. Always do a patch test on your ski before applying it to bigger areas of your body.

Shop Now

4. Green Tea.

Green tea is a valuable natural ingredient in antioxidant skin car due to its anti-inflammatory properties. It is a good rosacea therap because it contains polyphenols, which assist in relieving symptom including burning, itching, and redness.

Green tea may be consumed as a herbal supplement or applied topi cally via lotions, moisturizers, and serums. Osmosis Replenish MD Antioxidant Infusion Serum includes 17 antioxidants, including gree tea extract.

op now.

oatmeal

Oatmeal is an effective home therapy for rosacea. It strengthens the ter skin layer, reduces irritation, and prevents moisture loss. Ground t kernels, often known as colloidal oatmeal, may smooth and soothe itated skin, as well as reduce rashes and burns.

oose products containing colloidal oatmeal, such as ZO Skin Health ydrating Creme. Alternatively, you may make a DIY face mask at me by mixing a few tablespoons of oats with water.

op Now:

Lavender.

Lavender oil has soothing properties that may help soothe skin ritations, reduce itching and dryness, and treat symptoms of disorders ch as rosacea, eczema, and psoriasis. Its antifungal and antimicrobial mponents, including as linalool, geraniol, and eucalyptol, consider- ly reduce stress-induced flare-ups and give relief.

se diluted lavender essential oil in small amounts to treat the inflamed ea, or put a few drops into your favorite moisturizer for calming fects.

Niacinamide

Niacinamide is a B3 vitamin that is required for proper skin health. s strong antioxidant properties assist in reducing acne, eczema, and osacea-related redness, swelling, and blotchiness. Rosacea affects all kin types, but niacinamide is particularly beneficial for oily skin since controls sebum production and reduces excessive oiliness.

Niacinamide is commonly added to creams and lotions for topic application. To decrease skin flushing, use a moisturizer with niacinamide.

Niacin is another kind of vitamin B3 that promotes skin health an may be increased with vitamin B IV therapy.

8. Comfrey

This plant's roots contain allantoin and rosmarinic acid, which m help reduce edema, puffiness, and irritation. These calming chemica neutralize free radicals, protect the skin from external stresses, an relieve the burning sensation caused by rosacea.

Comfrey extracts are used in ointments, lotions, and salves to tre redness, itching, and irritation. Cosmetic products containing natur comfrey or allantoin can help speed up the healing process.

9. Burdock

Burdock is a popular plant extract used to lighten and tone the ski According to studies, its seed extract improves blood circulation an skin brightness.

The root is known as a "blood purifier" in traditional Chinese medicin because of its ability to fight germs and illness. Its powerful antibacteri and antioxidant properties help to control rosacea symptoms whil protecting the skin from oxidative stress.

Burdock is available in three forms: herbal supplements, fresh root, an seed extract.

10. feverfew

Feverfew is a medicinal herb that has several health advantages, including migraine treatment. When applied to the skin, this so-called medieval aspirin" possesses powerful antibacterial qualities. Its strong anti-inflammatory properties aid in alleviating rosacea symptoms.

Feverfew also protects the skin from ultraviolet (UV) radiation and other environmental stresses that might injure it.

Only use topical feverfew products that are devoid of parthenolides, since they might cause skin irritation (e.g., contact allergic dermatitis).

1. Raw honey.
Raw honey may help relieve pain, soothe the skin, and prevent flare-ups. It also helps to prevent dryness by locking in more moisture, relaxing the skin, and improving its barrier. According to one research, using high-quality kanuka honey on the skin may help with rosacea symptoms.

You may apply a tiny amount of pure kanuka or manuka honey straight to your skin, or use a topical solution containing the finest raw honey, such as iS Clinical Warming Honey Cleanser.

iS Clinical's Warming Honey Cleanser for Rosacea.
  Shop Now

2. Turmeric
This root includes antioxidants derived from curcumin, a bioactive compound with significant anti-inflammatory and wound-healing effects. It helps with painful or irritated rosacea symptoms, acne scarring, and psoriasis.

You may use it in topical treatments, make a poultice by combining turmeric powder and water, or apply a little amount of essential turmeric oil diluted in a carrier oil. Turmeric may leave a yellow tint, so apply sparingly to prevent coloring your skin.

13. Tea Tree Oil.

Tea tree oil has calming ingredients that reduce irritation and inflammation. Although it is not a typical therapy for rosacea, one research found that tea tree oil gel reduces inflammation and redness in rosacea patients.

It also functions as a natural antibacterial, treating open wounds and hastening wound healing. Its anti-fungal and antibacterial characteristics aid to reduce skin irritation and remove infections.

It may be diluted with a carrier oil and applied straight to the skin.

14. Cucumber

Cucumber has a cooling action that soothes irritated skin and alleviates the feeling of burning. It also moisturizes the skin and lowers swelling, bringing relief and comfort.

Cucumbers are high in anti-inflammatory vitamins C, beta carotene, and manganese, which help protect the skin from free radicals. Cucumber contains antioxidants, which assist in eliminating blemishes and lessen the look of redness associated with rosacea.

You may buy cucumber extract-based products or create your own calming mask with fresh cucumber and other natural components appropriate for your skin type.

ote that cucumbers aren't the sole option to nurture your skin. Vitamin C IV treatment may also help enhance antioxidants and detoxify your skin, resulting in better skin health.

5. Licorice extract.

Licorice root is one of the oldest herbal treatments that may be used topically. Its main active ingredients, glycyrrhizin, coumarins, and flavonoids, have multiple antioxidant, antibacterial, and antiviral qualities that decrease redness and soothe the skin.

Licorice extract is often used to treat eczema and acne, but it may also help with secondary skin concerns caused by rosacea, such as pigmentation or flushing.

You may include licorice extract in your skincare routine by selecting products that contain this natural cure.

6. Probiotics and prebiotics.

Poor gut health may cause or exacerbate rosacea symptoms. A well-balanced diet high in probiotics and prebiotics promotes intestinal health and improves skin condition.

Probiotics are "good" bacteria that help your digestive system. They are often found in fermented foods like kefir and yogurt. Prebiotics are high-fiber meals that nourish the beneficial microorganisms in your stomach. Prebiotic foods include garlic, onions, chia seeds, and almonds.

There are also a number of supplements that may assist improve gut health. We propose Vibrant Biome or Vibrant Digest, which may help minimize redness by promoting healthy gastrointestinal bacteria.

17. Acupuncture.

Acupuncture is a traditional Chinese medical technique that involve putting small needles into the body to increase energy flow. Th approach may alleviate the redness, irritation, and flushing associate with rosacea.

Acupuncture offers brief relief. To get the best effects, supplemer the therapy with prescribed herbs and lifestyle adjustments (such a avoiding hot and spicy foods).

A holistic facial is a natural treatment option for rosacea.

18. Holistic facials

Holistic facials involve acupressure and lymphatic drainage massag using essential oils and natural plant components. These method promote circulation and enhance toxin removal, reducing rosace symptoms.

Each treatment incorporates unique plant-based products and method customized to your skin type and condition. The Remedy Facial from Vibrant Skin Bar helps to reverse skin sensitivity and irritation and i particularly good for inflamed skin.

Buy Now, Use Later.

19. Lifestyle Changes

To manage your rosacea symptoms, try the following lifestyle changes

Use mild skincare products that have natural components.

Consume a balanced diet heavy in fiber, probiotics, and anti-inflammatory foods.

Avoid alcoholic beverages to minimize flushing.

Lower your cortisol levels by participating in stress-relieving activities.

Keep a food log to check if you have food intolerances.

Wear a broad-spectrum sunscreen to prevent UV-induced flare-ups.

When Should You Go to a Dermatologist?

Rosacea may grow to a chronic condition if left untreated. Some individuals benefit from over-the-counter treatment, while others require prescription medication.

Seek experienced medical treatment if you face any of the following:

After several weeks of consistent use, none of the natural cures give alleviation for your concerns.

The flare-ups get more frequent, and the symptoms worsen.

The skin texture changes (for example, it thickens or develops pimples).

The skin becomes irritated or develops an allergic reaction.

Other health problems or medications worsen this skin condition.

Conclusion

Natural rosacea treatments are easy at-home solutions that might help you manage your symptoms. They are simple and cost-effective options for individuals who choose natural remedies over harsh chemicals.

However, natural remedies are not always effective and may result in unforeseen effects. Consult a qualified dermatologist for more information and help.

III

Part Three

A Guide for Exercising, What to Eat to Avoid Rosacea Flares, and 7 Things to Pack in Your Beach Bag if You're Managing Rosacea

Chapter 9

A Guide to Exercise while Managing Rosacea.

Intense exercise is a typical cause of rosacea flares, yet physical activity has several health and skin advantages. Here's how to get started without making things worse.

Even if you understand the advantages of regular exercise, you may avoid it for fear of aggravating your rosacea symptoms. Susan Bard, MD, a board-certified general and procedural dermatologist at Vive Dermatology in Brooklyn, New York, feels your worries are valid.

Rosacea is a disorder in which blood vessel instability causes flushing and blushing. "When we exercise, these unstable vessels dilate further, resulting in even more flushing," she advises.

According to a poll published in the Spring 2013 edition of Rosacea Review, a National Rosacea Society (NRS) publication, more than 80% of rosacea patients reported skin irritation when exercising.

Overexertion may exacerbate rosacea symptoms including redness, edema, and pimples, but it should not be avoided.

The point is that not getting enough exercise might have an impact o
your rosacea treatment as well as your general health.

Tsippora Shainhouse, MD, a board-certified dermatologist in Sant
Monica, California, believes that exercise has various advantage
including higher endorphins and lower stress, which aid in calming th
mind. "Stress is one trigger for rosacea flares, so stress reduction can b
a beneficial, long-term rosacea management technique, even if it cause
some temporary flushing due to the acute vasodilation."

Dr. Shainhouse goes on to explain how exercise distributes oxygenate
blood and nutrients throughout the body, including the skin, to rebuil
and repair cells. This may result in healthier-looking skin.

According to the aforementioned NRS research, 62 percent of respor
dents said that small workout program alterations reduced exercise
related pain.

Rather than avoiding exercise altogether, discover how to modify you
routine to reduce the redness produced by a rosacea flare.

6 Do's and Don'ts of Working Out with Rosacea.

These rosacea care exercises may help you to live an active lifestyle
while minimizing your chances of a flare.

1. Avoid high-intensity activity if you don't want to cause a flare
   Although a recent research published in March 2017 in the journal

Med Research International discovered that high-intensity exercise d cardiovascular advantages, Dr. Bard warns that this kind of activity a frequent cause of rosacea flares. Shainhouse agrees. "High-intensity orkouts increase blood flow and heart rate temporarily, which can ke the skin appear more red in patients who already have vasodilation sociated with rosacea," according to the dermatologist.

e good news is that you may still fulfill the 2018 federal activity idelines by engaging in at least 150 minutes of moderate-intensity ercise each week, such as cycling, brisk walking, or housework, and minutes of high-intensity exercise. "Lower-intensity workouts won't ake your face flush as much," Shainhouse explains. The recommen- tions also recommended that you perform strength training at least ice a week.

Instead of lengthy training sessions, use brief bursts of action. Rather of conducting a continuous 45-minute exercise, the NRS ggests taking 15-minute breaks throughout the day. You'll continue benefit while lowering your chances of overheating and skin redness. this isn't feasible, switch between "hot" and "cool" activities. Spend 15 inutes exercising weights or doing aerobics, followed by stretching or wimming laps in the pool. Once you've calmed down, you may resume eightlifting or aerobics.

Do not let your body overheat. Wearing too many garments when exercising may cause heat. The merican Academy of Dermatology suggests wearing appropriate xercise clothing and layering it, removing it as needed. To remain ool, the NRS suggests wrapping a cold cloth over your neck or rubbing n ice cube on your skin. "Drinking cold water and keeping a cool cloth r spray bottle by your cardio machine to place on your face and neck

intermittently will help constrict blood vessels and reduce the ext
redness a little quicker," according to a news release that was given c
by the doctor's office.

**4. Exercise in the morning or evening, when the sun is not at i
peak.**

According to Shainhouse, the peak sun hours in the summer a
between 10 a.m. and 4 p.m., and those with rosacea are more vulnerat
to heat from UV rays than those without skin disease. This may promo
increased vasodilation and make the skin seem redder. If you lil
walking, jogging, bicycling, or trekking, do it in the early morning
evening. The National Recreation Service recommends looking f
covered routes and remembering to apply sunscreen.

5. Avoid exercising in stuffy environments.

Bard suggests keeping the environment air-conditioned to minimi
sweating when exercising inside. You may also generate a cross bree
by opening the windows or putting on a fan. Better still, turn to wate
"Consider swimming or water aerobics in a cool swimming pool instea
of working out on a stuffy indoor cardio machine or sweaty, enclose
spin studio," he went on to say.

6. Keep a water bottle handy to remain hydrated.

"The vessels in the skin vasodilate to help dissipate heat, but if you'r
dehydrated and can't sweat sufficiently, the body will not cool of
quickly and redness may persist for longer than you like," according t
the doctor. To avoid dehydration, the Mayo Clinic suggests drinkin
water before, during, and after exercise. This might assist your body
natural cooling system to work correctly.

The Last Word on Exercise and Rosacea Symptoms.

Keeping an activity record will help you determine which workouts are impacting your rosacea.

It is typical for your skin to get red after exercising. Do not allow self-consciousness to interfere with your fitness program.

While patients with rosacea may look a little pinker when exercising, and their skin may feel sensitive and irritated when the salty sweat sits on it, overall, exercise is healthy and should not be avoided because of this common skin condition," she went on to point out.

What Should I Eat To Avoid Rosacea Flares?

Rosacea is a chronic inflammatory skin disorder that mostly affects the mid-face. Symptoms vary; some people have facial redness or flushing. Some people have more visible blood vessels, red acne-like lesions on their faces, or thicker skin around their noses.

Once you've been diagnosed with this skin condition, your dermatologist will recommend medical treatment to relieve your symptoms. While numerous treatments may help with rosacea symptoms, Erum Ilyas, MD, a board-certified dermatologist in Philadelphia, feels that avoiding certain triggers is the most effective method to manage this chronic condition.

Rosacea triggers vary from person to person, but they may include heat, cold air, intense exercise, sun exposure, emotions and stress, and medication - anything that increases blood flow to the skin's surface. Certain foods may aggravate rosacea in certain people.

To be clear, eating does not "cause" rosacea. The specific etiology of this disease is unknown. However, some meals and components have been identified as triggers.

Which foods should you avoid if you have rosacea?

Spicy foods.

Spicy or spicy foods, whether added to recipes or craved for an extra kick, might be one of the numerous causes of rosacea flares.

Cayenne pepper, red pepper, black pepper, curry, paprika, and other spicy foods may dilate the tiny blood vessels under your skin, causing flushing.

Replace these spices with oregano, sage, and basil while cooking. These substances may provide the desired amount of flavor without causing skin irritation.

Alcohol

Avoiding alcohol may also help to alleviate rosacea symptoms. According to the National Rosacea Society, red wine has a greater risk of flares, although symptoms may also occur with bourbon, gin, vodka, champagne, and beer.

Alcohol causes blood vessels in the face to expand, increasing blood ow in the region.

ot drinks.
Some people cannot start their day without a cup of coffee. On a cool
ay, steaming tea or chocolate can quickly warm you up.

you have frequent rosacea flare-ups, eliminating hot beverages (which
crease blood flow to the face and induce flushing) may help to improve
e appearance of your skin.

his does not mean giving up coffee or tea; nevertheless, cooled coffee
r tea may be a better option.

igh-Histamine Foods
Fruits are rich in nutrients and antioxidants, yet some contain a lot
f histamine. This is an organic compound that triggers an immune
esponse. According to Dr. Ilyas, histamine causes vasodilation, or
lood vessel relaxation, which exacerbates or provokes rosacea flares.
When the blood vessels in the face dilate, redness develops.

Tomatoes, pineapple, strawberries, papaya, and red plums may all
rigger this reaction.

Keep in mind that fruits are not the only meals that might trigger
histamine release. Other triggers include eggplant, spinach, mushrooms,
hellfish, legumes, alcohol, and fermented foods (for example, aged
cheese).

Dairy items, such as yogurt, sour cream, and cheese, might be a trigger
for certain people.

Dairy has significant levels of vitamin D and calcium, but it may also promote inflammation. Inflammation may produce increased facial redness and puffiness.

Eliminating dairy from your diet may help reduce rosacea redness and symptoms. It's easier said than done, but if you can't completely eliminate dairy, try to restrict it. Replace cow's milk with rice, almond or soymilk. Look for dairy-free options including ice cream, yogurt and cheese.

Chocolate

Giving up chocolate may scare you. However, chocolate may irritate rosacea in some people because to the presence of cinnamaldehyde, the molecule that gives cinnamon its flavor. It might dilate blood vessels causing the skin to flush.

Strategies to Identify Your Rosacea Triggers

It may be difficult to tell which foods cause rosacea. Ilyas recommends keeping a "month-at-a-glance" calendar to track your food consumption and the worst days for rosacea flare-ups.

"Many of my patients note early-in-the-week flares, sometimes triggered by red wine with a weekend dinner," she went on to say.

"If your rosacea flares up early in the week but fades later, focus on your weekend activities. However, if the week starts well but your skin deteriorates over the week, return to your normal weekday regimen."

As you review your food diary, you may discover that particular foods

gger flares, or you may conclude that food has no influence on your
ndition.

hat Foods Can Help You with Rosacea?

ertain foods may aggravate rosacea by causing an inflammatory
sponse, whilst others can help your body fight inflammation and
lieve symptoms.

day doesn't go by where I'm not asked what role inflammatory
ods play in various skin conditions," Ilyas was quoted as saying.
ome studies have linked an increased incidence of gastrointestinal
oblems and bacterial overgrowth in our stomachs to rosacea flare-
s. Similarly, a high-fiber [prebiotic] diet may reduce flare-ups and
flammation.

yas classifies prebiotic fibers as onions, raw garlic, bananas, endive,
paragus, and whole grains.

ods strong in omega-3 fatty acids may help to lower inflammatory
oteins in the body, hence alleviating rosacea eye symptoms.

2016 study monitored 130 ocular rosacea patients who were given
ietary omega-3 fatty acids for six months. Symptoms included a gritty
nsation, itching, burning, and red eyes. After six months, the people
ported that their vision problems had greatly improved.

addition to supplements, omega-3-rich meals include wild salmon,
na, sardines, mackerel, walnuts, chia seeds, and flaxseeds.

Final remarks on the Rosacea Diet Plan.

Identifying rosacea triggers requires work, but keeping track everything you eat and drink, as well as recording your symptom may help you uncover troublesome products.

If you suspect that food is to blame, an exclusion diet might provi proof. Stop eating a certain meal for a set length of time to see if yo symptoms improve, and then reintroduce it to see if they return.

Chapter 10

Items to Pack in Your Beach Bag If You Have Rosacea.

Sunshine is one of the most common triggers for a flare-up, but you don't have to spend the entire summer indoors. Here's how you may prepare for the next beach days.

Summer provides beautiful weather and fun activities, but it also increases the likelihood of flares for those with rosacea. Why? "The sun is one of the most common triggers of rosacea, period," says Kenneth Mark, MD, a board-certified cosmetic dermatologist in New York City and Aspen.

Unfortunately, that's not all. According to Ayelet Mizrachi-Jonisch, MD, a dermatologist in Katonah, New York, heat and humidity, which are common during the summer, can be uncomfortable. A survey published in Rosacea Review, the National Rosacea Society's newsletter, found that almost all of the 739 respondents tried to reduce the likelihood of rosacea flares caused by the sun and heat, with 88 percent claiming that these methods worked.

According to the American Academy of Dermatology (AAD), a flare may cause skin to flush for hours after you've been out of the sunlight. According to Dr. Mark, this can be mild, accompanied by pimples and pustules, or severe, resulting in full-blown red, sensitive, and painful cystic lesions.

It is critical to avoid flares because they exacerbate and prolong rosacea flushing over time. "Treatments which have worked in the past may become ineffective, and rosacea may progress and involve other areas of the skin," the dermatologist said. "Repeated flushing events may lead to permanent reddening of the skin."

As a result, trying to avoid flares is a wise decision. That doesn't mean you can't have fun this summer; just make sure you have these basics on hand before heading out for a day in the sun.

1. Pack a hat to shield your face from the sun.

To reduce the possibility of a flare, avoid exposing your face to as much sunlight as possible. Mizrachi-Jonisch believes that a broad-brimmed hat is appropriate. Don't only wear hats to the beach. The AAD suggests wearing one whenever you venture outside. Holding your hat up to the sun is an excellent way to check if it provides enough coverage. If you can't see direct light through the material, it still provides enough SPF protection.

2. Bring an umbrella for full-body covering at the beach.

The golden rule for managing rosacea on the beach is to seek shade whenever possible. If the beach you're visiting doesn't provide umbrellas, Mizrachi-Jonisch suggests carrying your own and staying under it as much as possible, especially during the warmest portion of the day.

Use a broad-spectrum sunscreen with at least SPF 30.

The AAD advises that people with rosacea use sunscreen every day, not only during the summer. Make it a broad-spectrum sunscreen with a minimum SPF of 30. Mineral sunscreens containing just titanium dioxide, zinc oxide, or both are suitable for those with rosacea and sensitive skin. The National Rosacea Society recommends using sunscreen 30 minutes before leaving the house so that it may fully penetrate. Next, reapply every two hours, or more often if you work out or swim.

. Carry a water bottle to avoid dehydration, which may exacerbate Rosacea symptoms.

Mizrachi-Jonisch believes that staying hydrated is critical for controlling flares, so she recommends bringing a large water bottle to the beach. Dehydration poses a health issue because "when we are dehydrated, both our mucous membranes and skin are also dehydrated, and dry skin has decreased barrier function, which can set off an inflammatory cascade and thus trigger rosacea flares," Mark said.

. Prefer fresh, anti-inflammatory meals over stimulating ones.

According to research, rosacea has a gut-skin connection, with hot and spicy foods being common triggers. According to Mizrachi-Jonisch, some rosacea patients have discovered that eating anti-inflammatory foods can help them manage their condition. Her main point is that foods that are good for your health—fruits, vegetables, and whole grains—also benefit your skin. Bring some fruits and vegetables to snack on throughout your beach day. Mark recommends fruits and vegetables, such as broccoli.

. Use a spray bottle filled with cold water to stay cool in the sun.

According to the Cleveland Clinic, hot outdoor temperatures can cause your skin to flush, so stay cool, even in the shade. One approach is to bring a spray bottle with you. Fill it with cold water before leaving the house, then use it to cool your face whenever you feel hot.

7. Continue taking your Rosacea medication to keep your symptoms under control.

Mizrachi-Jonisch recommends carrying your rosacea medication with you at all times, especially during the warmer months when you spend time outside. When a flare appears, it is critical to act quickly. "The sooner a flare is treated and prevented from exacerbating, the easier it is to treat," he went on to say. The National Rosacea Society recommends that you continue to take your medication because long-term treatment is likely the most effective way to avoid complications